Table of Contents

PREVIEW

End-stage renal disease, also called end-stage kidney disease or kidney failure, occurs when chronic kidney disease — the gradual loss of kidney function — reaches an advanced state. In end-stage renal disease, your kidneys no longer work as they should to meet your body's needs.

Your kidneys filter wastes and excess fluids from your blood, which are then excreted in your urine. When your kidneys lose their filtering abilities, dangerous levels of fluid, electrolytes and wastes can build up in your body.

With end-stage renal disease, you need dialysis or a kidney transplant to stay alive. But you can also choose to opt for conservative care to manage your symptoms — aiming for the best quality of life during your remaining time.

Kidney disease can affect your body's ability to clean your blood, filter extra water out of your blood, and help control your blood pressure. It can also affect red blood cell production and vitamin D metabolism needed for bone health.

You're born with two kidneys. They're on either side of your spine, just above your waist.

When your kidneys are damaged, waste products and fluid can build up in your body. That can cause swelling in your ankles, nausea, weakness, poor sleep, and shortness of breath. Without treatment, the damage can get worse and your kidneys may eventually stop working. That's serious, and it can be life-threatening.

RENAL DIET RECIPES

BREAKFAST

1. Instant Pot Beef Bourguignon
Prep Time: 25 Minutes

Cook Time: 3hrs 2 Minutes

Servings: 8

Ingredients

- 8 slices bacon cut into ¼-inch slices
- 1 tbsp. canola oil
- 1 3 – pound boneless beef chuck fat removed and cut into 1½-inch cubes
- Kosher salt
- Freshly ground black pepper
- 5 carrots sliced diagonally into 1-inch chunks
- 1 large yellow onion diced
- 4 cloves garlic minced; divided
- 2 tbsp. all-purpose flour
- 1 750 ml bottle good red wine such as Pinot Noir or Cote du Rhone
- ½ cup cognac
- 1 2 – cup can beef broth
- 1 tbsp. 1 tablespoon tomato paste
- 1 tbsp. fresh thyme leaves or ½ teaspoon dried)
- 1 bay leaf
- 4 tbsp. unsalted butter
- 1 pound frozen pearl onions thawed

- 1 pound fresh cremini mushrooms stems or mashed potatoes removed and caps thickly sliced

Instructions

1. Heat oven to 325°F
2. Pat the beef dry with paper towels, season with salt & pepper; set aside.
3. In a small bowl, combine the flour, salt and pepper; set aside.
4. Add the bacon to a Dutch oven set over medium heat. Cook until the fat has rendered and use a slotted spoon to transfer the bacon pieces to a paper towel-lined plate.
5. beef burgundy recipe
6. Add 1-tablespoon canola oil to the pot and wait 30 seconds to allow the oil to heat. Add about ⅓rd. beef cubes to the pot, turning as needed, to sear all sides. Repeat with remaining beef searing ⅓rd. of the beef at-a-time. Transfer the beef to the same plate with the bacon.
7. Add the carrots and chopped onions to the Dutch oven. Sprinkle with 1-teaspoon kosher salt and ½ teaspoon freshly ground black pepper. Cook 8-12 minutes or until the vegetables have lightly browned. Add half the minced garlic and cook another 30 seconds.
8. Add the beef and bacon back to the pot with the vegetables and mix. Sprinkle flour over the meat/vegetable mixture and cook, stirring often, for 5 minutes.
9. Add the wine slowly while deglazing (scraping the flavorful bits) the pan. Add the cognac and enough beef broth to almost cover the meat.
10. Add the tomato paste, thyme leaves and bay leaf and stir. Bring back to a simmer, cover the pot with a tight-fitting lid and place it in the oven.

11. Cook the beef 2-3 hours, stirring occasionally, until the meat is fork-tender.
12. While the beef cooks, prepare the onions & mushrooms. Heat 2 tablespoons butter in a medium saucepan over medium-low heat. Add the thawed pearl onions and season with kosher salt and freshly ground black pepper. Cook until the onions are lightly browned on all sides, 8-10 minutes. Add the remaining 2 tablespoons butter, sliced cremini mushrooms and the remaining minced garlic to the pan. Cook until golden brown, about 6-8 minutes. Season to taste with kosher salt and freshly ground black pepper, if needed. Set aside until beef is ready.
13. When the beef is cooked through and tender, transfer the stew from the oven to the stovetop. Remove the lid and set the burner to medium heat. Add the pearl onion/mushroom mixture and bring the stew to a boil (stovetop). Reduce the temperature to low and simmer 15 minutes. Remove the stew from the heat and let sit another 15 minutes.
14. Discard the bay leaf and rosemary sprig.
15. Season the stew to taste, and serve over mashed potatoes (or mushrooms) or egg noodles.
16. Instant pot Beef bourguignon with mushrooms
17. Enjoy as you lick your plate clean!

2. Homemade Pizza Casserole

Prep Time: 25 Minutes

Cook Time: 45 Minutes

Servings: 7

Ingredients

- 1 tbsp. Ghee or other fat
- 1½ lbs. Ground pork sausage casing removed
- 2 cups Sliced mushrooms
- 1 tbsp. Olive oil
- Pinch of sea salt
- 1 cup Pizza sauce
- 2 Plum tomatoes diced
- 2 tbsp. Basil leaves sliced
- 1 cup Mozzarella Cheese shredded
- 2 oz. Pepperoni slices

Instructions

1. Preheat oven to 400 degrees; grease an 8 x 8 casserole dish with ghee and set aside.
2. Over medium heat, cook sausage in a large skillet, making sure to break sausage into small pieces.
3. While sausage is cooking, in a small saucepan over medium low heat, combine pizza sauce, diced tomatoes and basil. Cook until sauce is heated.
4. Once sausage is cooked, place meat on a layer of paper towels to drain. Wipe skillet clean and heat olive oil over medium heat. Once oil is hot add in mushrooms

and sprinkle with a pinch of salt. Sauté until browned, softened and excess water removed.

5. Place the sausage in the casserole dish, making sure it is spread evenly. Next top sausage with mushrooms. Add sauce, spreading evenly on top. Sprinkle cheese on top of sauce and then layer on the pepperoni.

6. Bake for 20-25 minutes, until cheese is melted. Serve immediately.

3. Caramel Apple Lasagna
Prep Time: 10 Minutes

Cook Time: 20 Minutes

Servings: 8

Ingredients

- 1 pouch (17.5 ounces) oatmeal cookie mix + ingredients required on the pouch
- ½ cup butter, melted
- 8 ounces cream cheese, softened
- 1 cup powdered sugar
- ½ cup + 2 tablespoons caramel sauce
- 12 ounces cool whip, thawed
- 2 cups apple pie filling
- 2 boxes vanilla instant pudding
- 3 cups cold milk

Instructions

1. Preheat oven to 375 degrees. Bake cookies according to package directions, then cool completely.I
2. In a food processor, blitz half the baked cookies until they become coarse crumbs. Transfer to a medium bowl, then continue blitzing the remaining half of cookies to coarse crumbs and add to the bowl. Mix in the melted butter until well-combined. Press the cookie mixture evenly into the bottom of a 9×13 baking dish, then set aside.
3. In a mixing bowl, beat together the cream cheese, powdered sugar, and ½ cup of the caramel sauce with

a hand mixer until smooth. Gently fold in 2 cups of the Cool Whip until well-combined, then spread evenly over the prepared crust. Top evenly with the apple pie filling.

4. In another mixing bowl, beat together the pudding mixes and milk for about 2 minutes, or until thick. Scoop over the apple layer, spreading evenly, then spread the remaining Cool Whip over. Cover and chill 4 hours.

5. When ready to serve, slice into squares and drizzle caramel sauce on top. Enjoy!

4. Beef Burgundy
Prep Time: 25 Minutes

Cook Time: 2hrs 2 Minutes

Servings: 7

Ingredients

- 2 tablespoons olive oil
- 2 pounds beef chuck roast cut into small pieces
- 2 cups beef broth
- 1 ½ cups dry red wine
- 1 teaspoon salt
- ½ teaspoon dried thyme crushed
- ¼ teaspoon ground black pepper
- 2 ½ cups sliced fresh mushrooms
- 3 onions sliced

Instructions

1. To begin, heat some oil in the Dutch oven over medium-high heat.
2. Once the oil is hot, add the beef cubes and cook until they are browned on all sides.
3. Add onions, mushrooms, carrots, celery, garlic, and thyme to the pot and cook until the vegetables have softened.
4. Next add red wine to deglaze the pot and then add beef broth, tomato paste and bay leaves.
5. Simmer everything together for 1-2 hours or until the meat is tender. Serve with your favorite variations to complete this delicious meal!

5.Antipasto Skewers
Prep Time: 25 Minutes

Cook Time: 00 Minutes

Servings: 6

Ingredients

- 10 bocconcini cocktail sized
- 10 cherry tomatoes
- 10 pitted olives
- 10 marinated artichokes
- 10 slices roasted red pepper about 1" each
- 20 slices salami or substitute half for Mortedella
- balsamic reduction & fresh basil and parsley for garnish optional

Instructions

1. Start by threading the ingredients onto wooden skewers in an alternating pattern. (If you're using wooden skewers, make sure to soak them in water for at least 30 minutes before use so they don't burn when cooking)
2. Once all the ingredients are on the skewers, drizzle with olive oil and sprinkle with salt and pepper to taste.
3. Place the skewers on a baking sheet and bake in a preheated oven at 375 degrees Fahrenheit for 15-20 minutes or until the cheese is melted and bubbly.

4. Serve them warm with some crusty bread or crackers on the side for an impressive appetizer that your guests will love!

6. Korean Pickled Garlic
Prep Time: 15 Minutes

Cook Time: 5 Minutes

Servings: 3

Ingredients

- 1 cup peeled garlic cloves
- 1 cup rice vinegar
- 1/4 cup sugar
- 1 tablespoon salt
- 1/4 teaspoon black pepper
- 2 dried red peppers optional or Korean red chili flakes (gochugaru) – 1 teaspoon (optional)
- 1/2 onion thinly sliced (optional)

Instructions

1. In a small saucepan, combine the rice vinegar, sugar, salt, black pepper, and dried red peppers (if using). Bring the mixture to a boil over medium-high heat, stirring until the sugar and salt dissolve.
2. Reduce the heat to low and simmer the mixture for 5 minutes, then remove it from the heat and let it cool to room temperature.
3. In a clean glass jar or container, add the peeled garlic cloves and sliced onions (if using). Pour the cooled vinegar mixture over the garlic and onions, making sure they are fully submerged.
4. Cover the jar or container with a lid and let it sit at room temperature for 1-2 days to allow the flavors to

develop. After that, store it in the refrigerator for up to a month or so. The longer it sits, the more flavorful it becomes!

7. Creamy chicken wild rice soup
Prep Time: 10 Minutes

Cook Time: 40 Minutes

Servings: 6

Ingredients

- 2 tbsp. butter
- 1 pound Mushrooms (sliced)
- 1 tbsp. butter
- 1 onion (diced)
- 2 carrots (diced)
- 2 stalks celery (diced)
- 2 cloves garlic (chopped)1
- 1 tbsp. thyme (chopped)
- 6 cups chicken broth
- 1 cup wild rice (or a blend of rice including wild rice)
- 1½ cups chicken, cooked and diced or shredded
- 1 cup milk or cream
- 1 cup parmigianoreggiano (parmesan)
- grated salt and pepper to taste

Instructions

1. Melt the butter in a pan over medium-high heat, add the mushrooms and cook until the mushrooms have released their liquids and the liquid has evaporated, about 10-15 minutes, before setting aside.
2. butter and mushroom in the preparation of chicken wild rice soup

3. Melt the butter in the pan, add the onions, carrots and celery and cook until tender, about 8-10 minutes.
4. Mix in the garlic and thyme and cook until fragrant, about a minute.
5. Add the broth, rice, chicken and mushrooms, bring to a boil, reduce the heat and simmer, covered, until the rice is tender, about 20-30 minutes.
6. mushroom, chicken and rice
7. Mix in the milk and cheese and cook until the cheese has melted, before seasoning with salt and pepper to taste.

8. Cantonese Pork Brain Omelette
Prep Time: 25 Minutes

Cook Time: 30 Minutes

Servings: 8

Ingredients

- 4 pork brains cleaned and diced
- 4 eggs
- 1/4 cup milk
- 1/4 cup chopped onions
- 1/4 cup chopped bell peppers
- 2 cloves minced garlic
- 1/2 tsp salt
- 1/4 tsp black pepper
- 2 tbsp vegetable oil

Instructions

1. In a medium-sized mixing bowl, beat the eggs and milk together until well combined. Set aside.
2. eggs for making pork brain omelette
3. In a large skillet, heat the vegetable oil over medium-high heat.
4. Add the diced pork brains to the skillet and cook until they are lightly browned on all sides, stirring occasionally.
5. Add the chopped onions, bell peppers, and garlic to the skillet and continue cooking until the vegetables are tender and fragrant.

6. Pour the egg mixture into the skillet, making sure to distribute it evenly over the pork brain and vegetable mixture.
7. a mixture of eggs and pork brain omelette
8. Season the omelette with salt and black pepper, then use a spatula to gently lift the edges of the omelette and allow the uncooked eggs to flow underneath.
9. Continue cooking the omelette until the eggs are fully cooked and the omelette is set, flipping it over once halfway through cooking.
10. Slide the omelette onto a plate and serve hot. Garnish the omelette with chopped scallions or cilantro, or serve it with a side of steamed rice or stir-fried vegetables.

9. Raclette Cheese Wheel

Prep Time: 25 Minutes

Cook Time: 5 Minutes

Servings: 6

Ingredients

- Semi-hard cheese (raclette)
- Potatoes (boiled and sliced into thin rounds)
- Pickles
- Cured meat

Instructions

1. Choose the right equipment: To melt raclette cheese, you will need a special raclette grill or a pan with a melting tray. The melting tray is placed under the heating element, and the cheese is placed in the tray. The cheese will melt slowly, and you can scrape it onto your plate with a spatula.
2. Prepare the cheese: Before melting the raclette cheese, you need to prepare it. Remove the rind from the cheese wheel and slice the cheese into thin slices. This allows the cheese to melt quickly and evenly.
3. Heat up the grill: If you are using a raclette grill, heat it up according to the manufacturer's instructions. If you are using a pan, heat it over medium heat until hot.
4. Melt the cheese: Once the grill or pan is hot, place the cheese slices in the melting tray. If you are using a raclette grill, place the tray under the heating element. If you are using a pan, place the tray on top of the pan.

5. Scrape the cheese: Once the cheese has melted, use a special raclette scraper or spatula to scrape the melted cheese onto a plate of food. The cheese will be gooey and delicious, perfect for pairing with boiled potatoes, crusty bread, and cured meats.

10. Butter Garlic Chicken

Prep Time: 10 Minutes

Cook Time: 30 Minutes

Servings: 4

Ingredients

- 3 tablespoons olive oil
- 1 1/2 pounds boneless skinless chicken breasts pounded to an even thickness (4-6 average-sized breasts)
- 1 teaspoon salt to taste
- 1 teaspoon freshly ground black pepper or to taste
- 1/2 cup white wine* or chicken broth or as necessary
- 3 tablespoons unsalted butter or more if you want extra sauce
- 1 tablespoon garlic finely minced; or to taste
- 2 teaspoons fresh parsley optional for garnishing

Instructions

1. To make the butter garlic marinade, mix together the butter and garlic in a small bowl until well-blended.
2. Add the black pepper, salt and pepper flakes to the mixture and stir to combine. You can add heavy cream if you like. Pour the mixture over the chicken pieces in a bowl or container and refrigerate for at least an hour.
3. Turn the chicken pieces occasionally while they are marinating to ensure they are evenly coated with the marinade.

4. To prepare the dish:
5. Heat your oven or slow cooker on low heat setting and add 2-3 tablespoons of olive oil to coat the bottom of a large baking dish with oil. Add 4-6 boneless skinless chicken breasts or thighs (about 1½ pound) to the baking dish and drizzle with half of the butter garlic marinade from earlier.
6. Season with salt and pepper to taste and spread out evenly across each piece of chicken. Bake at 350 degrees Fahrenheit for approximately 8 hours or until cooked through.
7. Make sure to flip the pieces of chicken over after 6 hours and add more butter garlic marinade if needed. Serve immediately with steamed rice if desired and enjoy!

LUNCH

11. Mushroom Spaghetti Squash
Prep Time: 15 Minutes

Cook Time: 45 Minutes

Servings: 5

Ingredients

- 8 ounces sliced cremini mushrooms
- 1/3 cup chopped dried shiitake mushrooms about 1 1/2 ounces
- 6 garlic cloves peeled
- 1/2 cup vegetable broth
- 2 1/2 pound spaghetti squash
- 1 Tablespoon olive oil
- Sea salt and black pepper
- 2 sprigs of fresh rosemary

Instructions

1. Start by preheating your oven to 375 degrees Fahrenheit.
2. Cut the spaghetti squash in half lengthwise and scooping out the seeds. Place the halves cut-side down on a baking sheet and roast them in the oven until tender (40-45 minutes)
3. While the squash is roasting, sauté a medley of mushrooms with garlic, onions, and herbs for added flavor. Once they are golden brown and fragrant, set them aside.

4. Once the spaghetti squash is cooked, use a fork to scrape out the flesh into strands that resemble spaghetti noodles. Combine them with the sautéed mushrooms for a delicious plant-based meal option that will satisfy even non-vegetarians.

12. Vegan Oreo Truffles
Prep Time: 20 Minutes

Cook Time: 00 Minutes

Servings: 25

Ingredients

- 1 packet vegan oreo cookies
- 1 8 oz package of vegan cream cheese softened
- 2 tbsp vegan margarine softened
- 12 ounces vegan chocolate chips
- 1 tbsp Coconut oil

Instructions

1. Crush the Oreo Cookies: Using a food processor or a plastic bag and a rolling pin, crush the Oreo cookies until they form a fine crumb texture. Reserve a small portion of the crushed cookies for decoration, if desired.
2. Combine the Ingredients: In a mixing bowl, combine the crushed Oreo cookies and the vegan cream cheese substitute or coconut cream. Mix well until the ingredients are fully incorporated and form a thick, dough-like consistency.
3. Shape the Truffles: Using a tablespoon or a small cookie scoop, portion out the dough and roll it into small, evenly sized balls. Place the truffles on a baking sheet lined with parchment paper.
4. Coat the Truffles: Dip each truffle into the melted vegan chocolate, ensuring it is fully coated. Use a fork

or a dipping tool to remove the truffle from the chocolate, allowing any excess to drip off. Place the coated truffles back onto the parchment-lined baking sheet.

5. Decorate (Optional): While the chocolate coating is still wet, sprinkle the tops of the truffles with the reserved crushed Oreo cookies, chopped nuts, cocoa powder, or sprinkles to add an extra touch of flavor and visual appeal.

6. Chill and Serve: Place the baking sheet with the coated truffles in the refrigerator for at least 30 minutes, or until the chocolate coating has set. Once chilled, the vegan Oreo truffles are ready to be served and enjoyed! Store any

13. Low Sodium Egg Salad
Prep Time: 00 Minutes

Cook Time: 20 Minutes

Servings: 16

Ingredients

- 8 eggs, straight from the refrigerator
- 1/2 cup of no salt added mayonnaise
- 2 teaspoons of salt-free stoneground mustard
- 1/4 teaspoon of onion powder
- 1/2 cup of celery, finely diced

For the No Salt Added Mayonnaise

- 1/4 cup of liquid egg substitute (ex: EggBeaters), at room temperature
- 2 1/2 tablespoons of distilled white vinegar
- 2/3 cup of canola oil (or neutral-flavored oil of your choice)

Instructions

1. Place the eggs in a single layer in a heavy saucepan and cover with cold water by at least one inch. Leaving the pot uncovered, turn the heat to high. As soon as the water comes to a boil, turn off the heat and cover. After 10 minutes, remove the cover and run cold water over the eggs for 1 minute. Set eggs aside to cool completely.
2. While your eggs are cooking, it is time to make your no salt added mayo. Place the egg substitute in a

medium-sized bowl. Add the vinegar and whisk until frothy. Note: you could use a hand blender or small food processor here if you prefer.

3. Very slowly, begin adding the oil in a thin stream while whisking continuously. If the oil starts to build up, stop pouring and whisk vigorously until it is incorporated. Continue adding the oil while whisking until all the oil has been used.
4. Set aside 1/2 cup of mayo for egg salad and refrigerate the extra.
5. Cut cool eggs in half, remove the yolks and place them into a medium-sized bowl. Chop the whites and set them aside.
6. Add no salt added mayo to the bowl of yolks and mash together until completely smooth.
7. Add mustard and onion powder. Stir until fully incorporated.
8. Fold in egg whites and celery.

14. Low Sodium Zucchini Bread

Prep Time: 10 Minutes

Cook Time: 45 Minutes

Servings: 10

Ingredients

- 3 eggs
- 1 cup of canola oil
- 1 cup of unsweetened applesauce
- 1 cup of sugar
- 2 teaspoons of vanilla extract
- 1 1/2 cups of all-purpose flour
- 1 1/2 cups of bread flour
- 2 teaspoons of no salt baking powder
- 1 tablespoon of ground cinnamon
- 2 cups of shredded zucchini

Instructions

1. Spray two 8x14 inch loaf pans with a non-stick spray that has flour. Preheat oven to 325 degrees.
2. In a large bowl, add flour, no salt baking powder, and cinnamon. Whisk together until mixed.
3. Beat eggs, oil, vanilla, applesauce, and sugar together by hand in a large bowl or using a stand mixer until everything is well combined.
4. Add dry ingredients to the creamed mixture and beat well.
5. Fold in zucchini until well combined. Pour batter into prepared pans.

6. Bake for 40 to 60 minutes, or until a tester inserted in the center comes out clean.
7. Cool in pan on a wire rack for about 20 minutes. Remove loaf and let cool completely on the rack before attempting to cut.

15.Low Sodium Chicken Salad
Prep Time: 5 Minutes

Cook Time: 45 Minutes

Servings: 6

Ingredients

- 1/2 cup of no-salt-added mayonnaise
- 1 cup of celery, finely chopped
- 4 hard-boiled eggs, chopped
- 1 teaspoon of no-salt-added lemon pepper
- 2 tablespoons of dried minced onion
- 1.5 pounds of cooked chicken, shredded

Instructions

To Cook The Chicken:

1. Rinse 1.5 pounds of boneless, skinless, chicken breasts thoroughly and place them in a large pot of unsalted water. Turn on the heat and bring it to a boil.
2. Reduce heat and simmer until chicken is done (about 45 minutes to an hour). When you are ready, remove the chicken from the pot and place it on a plate. With two forks, shred the chicken.

Assembling The Salad:

1. Put all ingredients - except mayonnaise - into a large bowl and toss together.
2. Add the no-salt-added mayo to the bowl and stir gently until everything is thoroughly mixed.
3. It is THAT simple!

16.Low Sodium Carrot Soup
Prep Time: 00 Minutes

Cook Time: 45 Minutes

Servings: 6

Ingredients

- 10 carrots, peeled and sliced
- 1 1/2 tablespoons of white granulated sugar
- 2 cups of water
- 3 tablespoons of all-purpose flour
- 1/4 teaspoon of ground black pepper
- 1/4 teaspoon of ground nutmeg
- 1 to 2 tablespoons of unsalted butter, to taste
- 4 cups of milk - do not use skim
- Fresh parsley for garnish

Instructions

1. In a Dutch oven or large saucepan, heat the carrots, sugar, and water until boiling. Cover and simmer on low until the carrots are very tender. This will take approximately 25 minutes.
2. Drain carrots from water. Reserve sugar water for later. Set aside.
3. In a separate saucepan over medium-high heat, whisk together flour, pepper, nutmeg, butter, and milk. Cook, stirring constantly until the white sauce thickens.

4. In a blender or food processor, add the cooked carrots and white sauce. Puree until smooth. See notes above regarding the pureeing process.
5. Slowly add sugar water until soup reaches desired consistency. Pour slowly! You don't want a watery soup on your hands.
6. Ladle into bowls and serve with parsley.

17. Low Sodium Apple Cranberry Stuffing

Prep Time: 1hr 30 Minutes

Cook Time: 40 Minutes

Servings: 6

Ingredients

- 2 cups of unsalted chicken broth
- 1 cup of dried cranberries
- 1/4 cup of unsalted butter
- 1 onion, chopped
- 1 bell pepper (red or green), chopped
- 1 cup of celery, chopped
- 2 Granny Smith apples, cored and finely chopped
- 3 large eggs
- 1/4 teaspoon of black pepper
- 1 (10.75 oz) can of unsalted cream of chicken soup
- 1/2 teaspoon ground cinnamon
- One 12-roll pack (about 8 cups) of King's Hawaiian Sweet Rolls

Instructions

1. Heat oven to 250 °F.
2. Cube the sweet rolls, spread out onto a large cookie or baking sheet.
3. Bake in 250-degree oven until bread is lightly toasted and completely dried out; about 60-90 minutes depending on your oven...be sure to stir the bread occasionally to ensure an even toasting.

4. With about 30 minutes left in your toasting process, take a small bowl and combine unsalted chicken broth and cranberries; let soak for at least 30 minutes.
5. When your breadcrumbs are done, remove from oven and increase oven temperature to 350 °F.
6. In a large skillet, melt butter over medium heat. Add onion, pepper and celery; cook for 5 minutes or until tender.
7. Add apples and cook for 5 minutes, stirring frequently.
8. Remove from heat and place in a large bowl.
9. In a separate bowl, beat 3 eggs with pepper. Set aside.
10. In the large bowl containing your cooked apples and vegetables, add the chicken broth/cranberry mixture, can unsalted cream of chicken soup, and cinnamon. Sitr until the condensed soup is completely incorporated.
11. Fold in toasted bread cubes, until bread is completely coated.
12. Add eggs and gently stir until combine Spoon mixture into prepared casserole dish and bake for 30 to 40 minutes or until center is set.

18. Low Sodium Pumpkin Cornbread Muffins
Prep Time: 35 Minutes

Cook Time: 00 Minutes

Servings: 12

Ingredients

- 1½ cups of all-purpose flour
- ½ cup of yellow cornmeal
- ½ cup of sugar
- 1½ teaspoons of salt-free baking powder
- ½ teaspoon of salt-free baking soda
- 1 teaspoon of ground cinnamon
- ½ teaspoon of nutmeg
- ¾ cup of canned pumpkin
- ½ cup of 1% buttermilk (see notes)
- ¼ cup of vegetable oil
- 2 large eggs, lightly beaten
- 1 teaspoon of pure vanilla extract
- Zest of 1 orange

Instructions

1. Preheat your oven to 350°F.
2. Spray a 12-cup muffin pan or 24-mini muffin pan with a nonstick spray that includes flour.
3. In a medium-sized bowl, add flour, cornmeal, sugar, baking powder, baking soda, and cinnamon. Whisk together.

4. In a separate medium-sized bowl, combine pumpkin, buttermilk, oil, eggs, vanilla, and orange zest. Stir until well combined.
5. Using a rubber spatula, fold the pumpkin mixture into the flour mixture until just combined. Don't overmix!
6. Using an ice cream or cookie scoop, spoon the batter into your prepared muffin pan.
7. Bake at 350 degrees in a preheated oven for about 20 minutes. Muffins are done when a toothpick inserted into the center of a muffin comes out clean.
8. Let muffins cool in the pan for 5 minutes. Pop muffins out onto a wire rack and let cool for another 10 minutes.

19. Low Sodium Chicken Divan
Prep Time: 10 Minutes

Cook Time: 35 Minutes

Servings: 10

Ingredients

- 1 can (10.5 ounce) of Campbell's Unsalted Cream of Chicken Soup
- 1 can (10.5 ounce) of Campbell's Unsalted Cream of Mushroom Soup
- 3/4 cup of sour cream
- 8 ounces of Swiss cheese, grated
- 1/4 cup of mayonnaise
- 1 teaspoon of curry powder
- 1/2 cup of unsalted chicken broth
- Half a lemon, juiced
- 2 packages (10 ounce) of frozen chopped broccoli, thawed, drained, and patted with paper towels
- 6 cups of cooked chicken, shredded or cubed
- 1 cup of Ritz Hint of Salt crackers
- 2 tablespoons of unsalted butter, melted

Instructions

1. Preheat the oven to 350 degrees.
2. Spray a 13x9 casserole dish with non-stick spray.
3. In a large mixing bowl, add both cans of unsalted soups, sour cream, Swiss cheese, curry powder, and mayonnaise. Gently mix together until well combined.

4. Add lemon juice and chicken broth. Stir until you have a smooth sauce.
5. Add broccoli and chicken. Mix well. Add to the prepared casserole dish.
6. Sprinkle crushed Ritz crackers over the chicken mixture and then drizzle melted butter over the crackers.
7. Bake in a 350-degree oven for 35 – 45 minutes, until hot and bubbly and the top is golden.

20. Low Sodium Penne alla Vodka

Prep Time: 10 Minutes

Cook Time: 40 Minutes

Servings: 7

Ingredients

- ¼ cup of olive oil
- 1½ cups of diced yellow onion
- ½ teaspoon of ground black pepper
- 1/8 teaspoon of crushed red pepper flakes
- 4 garlic cloves minced
- 1 cup of vodka
- 1 28 oz. can of no salt added crushed tomatoes
- 2 tablespoons of no salt added tomato paste
- 16 oz. box of penne pasta
- ½ cup of heavy whipping cream
- Chopped fresh parsley or basil for garnish

Instructions

1. Heat olive oil in a Dutch oven over medium heat; add onion, pepper, and red pepper flakes. Cook, stirring occasionally until softened, about 5 minutes.
2. Add garlic; cook, stirring occasionally, for about 2 minutes.
3. Add vodka; cook, stirring to release browned bits from the bottom of the pan.
4. Add tomatoes and tomato paste to the pan. Bring to a simmer; reduce heat to medium-low.

5. In a separate pot, cook pasta in unslated water per package directions for al dente.
6. Reserve 1 cup of pasta water; set aside. Drain pasta in a colander.
7. Remove tomato sauce from heat. Stir in cream until combined.
8. Add reserved pasta water, ¼ cup at a time, to emulsify the sauce if it's too thick. This is all about your personal preference, so you may not need all of the water.
9. Mix sauce and pasta in a large bowl. Garnish with parsley or basil if desired.

DINNER

21. Low Sodium Holiday Turkey with Pan Sauce
Prep Time: 20 Minutes

Cook Time: 4hrs 2 Minutes

Servings: 6

Ingredients

- 14-pound turkey
- 8 oz bottle of Westbrae Stoneground No Salt Added Mustard
- 8 oz jar of apricot preserves
- Pan Sauce
- 3/4 cup of unsalted chicken broth
- 1 1/2 tsp of corn starch
- 1/2 cup of a quality bourbon or apple cider
- 1 whole shallot, minced
- 2 tablespoons of unsalted butter

Instructions

Fully thaw your turkey following the directions on the packaging.

1. Preheat oven to 350°F.
2. Remove the giblets and neck from the turkey.
3. Fully rinse the turkey under cold water before placing it in a large roasting pan.
4. In a medium-sized mixing bowl, mix the bottle of mustard with the jar of apricot preserves. Make sure the two ingredients are thoroughly combined.

5. Gently lift the skin of the turkey to separate it from the body. Rub about one-third of the glaze under the skin of the turkey.
6. Using a sauce brush, coat the turkey with another third of the mustard apricot glaze. Make sure you don't forget the wings and legs!
7. Cover the remaining glaze and place it in the refrigerator. You'll need this in a couple of hours.
8. Cover the turkey with tin foil and roast in a 350-degree oven for approximately 4 hours. At the halfway point, apply a second coat of glaze to the outside of the bird using the remaining glaze.
9. Remove the foil for the last 30 minutes of baking to create a crisp crust.
10. Once the turkey has reached an internal temperature of 180°F as read by a meat thermometer, you can remove your turkey from the oven.
11. Your turkey needs to set for at least 15-20 minutes before you can carve it. Cut it up any sooner and you will lose all of the juice!
12. While the turkey is setting, use a turkey baster to collect drippings from the bottom of the roasting pan. Place these drippings into a saucepan.
13. Add shallots to the saucepan with drippings and saute over medium-high heat until shallots have softened.
14. Once shallots have softened, add bourbon or apple cider and bring to a low simmer. This is the point where we will cook off the alcohol.
15. As the pan is heating up, occasionally scrape the pan with a wooden spoon to incorporate all of the ingredients.
16. Continue to simmer until the liquid has reduced by about half.

17. Increase the heat to achieve a full simmer, whisk in the unsalted chicken stock, butter, and corn starch.
18. Allow the final liquid to reduce by half before pouring into a gravy boat or other similar serving container.

22. Low Sodium Cajun Chicken Pasta

Prep Time: 5 Minutes

Cook Time: 20 Minutes

Servings: 4

Ingredients

- 1/3 cup of low-fat milk
- 1 tablespoon of all-purpose flour
- 3 tablespoons of mascarpone cheese
- 2 teaspoons of salt-free Cajun season; see notes
- 1 teaspoon of garlic powder
- 8 ounces uncooked linguine (or spiral pasta)
- 1 pound chicken breast strips; cut into bite-sized pieces
- 1 cup unsalted chicken broth

Instructions

1. In a small blender make a slurry by combining milk, flour, and mascarpone cheese. Set aside.
2. Season chicken generously with Cajun seasoning and garlic powder.
3. Prepare pasta according to package directions.
4. Heat a large heavy nonstick skillet over medium-high heat; spray with cooking spray and add half of the chicken.
5. Sauté chicken for 5 to 6 minutes or until completely done, set aside on a plate and repeat with the remaining chicken. Set aside.

6. Reduce heat to medium-low; using the same skillet you used to cook the chicken add the chicken broth and the slurry mixture. Stir for about 2 minutes.
7. Return chicken to skillet and add cooked pasta; adjust Cajun seasoning to taste and toss well to coat.

23. Low Sodium Bourbon Glazed Carrots
Prep Time: 00 Minutes

Cook Time: 20 Minutes

Servings: 6

Ingredients

- 1 stick (8 tablespoons) of unsalted butter, sliced into 8 pieces
- 2 pounds of carrots, peeled and sliced into equal-sized pieces
- 1/2 cup of bourbon
- 1/3 cup of brown sugar
- 1 pinch of cayenne pepper (optional)
- Fresh ground pepper, to taste

Instructions

1. Using a thick-bottomed skillet, melt butter in a heavy skillet over medium heat.
2. Stir frequently. When butter foams up, add carrots. Stir until liquid evaporates from carrots and the carrots begin to brown around the edges. This will take around 6 minutes.
3. Reduce heat to medium-low and pour in the bourbon. Cook and stir until the bourbon is almost evaporated, this should take about 2-3 minutes.
4. Sprinkle in brown sugar. Stir until sugar is completely dissolved. Cook until carrots are almost cooked through, about 5 minutes.

5. When carrots are nearly tender, raise heat to medium-high to thicken the glaze, about 30-60 seconds.
6. Season with cayenne pepper and ground black pepper. Stir carrots and let simmer on low heat, uncovered, for about 5 minutes. This step is all about how soft you want your carrots. Like crisp carrots? Take them off the stovetop quickly. Like soft carrots? Leave them on longer.

24. Low Sodium Spicy Chicken Meatballs with Zucchini Noodles

Prep Time: 20 Minutes

Cook Time: 30 Minutes

Servings: 4

Ingredients

- 3 tablespoons of olive oil
- 2 tablespoons of Harissa (Moroccan red pepper sauce)
- 1 pound of zucchini, cut into noodles
- Sauce
- 4 cloves of garlic, crushed
- 2 large red bell peppers, chopped
- 1 teaspoon of olive oil
- 1/2 teaspoon of cumin
- 1/2 teaspoon of coriander
- 1/2 teaspoon of smoked paprika
- 1 teaspoon of crushed red pepper flakes
- 1/8 teaspoon ground black pepper
- Juice from 1/2 lemon

Chicken Meatballs

- 1 pound of ground chicken
- 1/2 yellow onion, chopped
- 1/2 cup of Panko breadcrumbs
- 3 cloves of minced garlic
- 1 large egg
- 1/2 teaspoon of smoked paprika
- 1 teaspoon of dried parsley

Instructions

1. Preheat oven to 425 degrees.
2. Spray a half sheet pan with olive oil and place chopped red bell peppers and crushed garlic cloves onto the pan. Bake at 425 for about 10 minutes. If you want a bit of char taste, turn your oven to broil the last few minutes to let your peppers brown. Watch the garlic! Do not let it burn.
3. Place peppers and garlic into a food processor or blender. Add olive oil, lemon juice, and all spices listed in the "sauce" section of the ingredients list and puree until you have a smooth sauce.
4. In a large mixing bowl, combine the meatball ingredients. Once thoroughly combined, roll into small to medium-sized meatballs. Whatever size you choose, keep it consistent. This will ensure an even cooking time for all your meatballs.
5. In a dutch oven, pour about three tablespoons of olive oil (enough to lightly coat the bottom of the pan) and warm over medium-high heat. Once the oil is hot, gently place your meatballs in the pan. Cook your meatballs for about 6 minutes, or until they are cooked to an internal temperature of 165 degrees. Be sure to turn your meatballs frequently to ensure you achieve a golden brown all over.
6. Once meatballs are cooked add your homemade sauce and the Moroccan red pepper sauce to the dutch oven. Stir until combined. Bring to a gentle boil, then reduce heat and simmer for 10 minutes.
7. Add your zucchini noodles and simmer for 3-4 minutes until the zucchini reaches a soft noodle-like texture.

25. No Sodium Flour Tortillas
Prep Time: 30 Minutes

Cook Time: 1 Minutes

Servings: 12

Ingredients

- 2 cups of all-purpose flour
- 1/4 cup olive oil (you'll want to use a light flavor)
- 3/4 cup warm water

Instructions

1. Combine ingredients in a bowl and stir together. Ultimately you will need to mix with your hands to ensure everything is fully incorporated. You don't want to see any specs of olive oil in your dough.
2. Knead your dough for about 10-15 minutes or until it is elastic enough to stretch without breaking.
3. Let dough rest for about 15 minutes to allow the gluten in the flour to relax which helps the tortilla to bubble while cooking. I put a damp paper towel over the dough to prevent it from drying out.
4. Tear apart your large dough ball into 12 equal size dough balls (a few less if you want larger tortillas).
5. Roll your dough balls into thin flat circles of equal size. Tip: if you roll the dough into a ball first, you are more likely to have a circular tortilla!
6. Place on hot griddle and cook for about 40 seconds, or until you get those nice classic air bubbles. Flip the tortilla and cook for an additional 20-30 seconds. The

exact time will depend on the thickness of your tortilla.

26. Low Sodium Zucchini Bread

Prep Time: 10 Minutes

Cook Time: 45 Minutes

Servings: 10

Ingredients

- 3 eggs
- 1 cup of canola oil
- 1 cup of unsweetened applesauce
- 1 cup of sugar
- 2 teaspoons of vanilla extract
- 1 1/2 cups of all-purpose flour
- 1 1/2 cups of bread flour
- 2 teaspoons of no salt baking powder
- 1 tablespoon of ground cinnamon
- 2 cups of shredded zucchini

Instructions

1. Spray two 8x14 inch loaf pans with a non-stick spray that has flour. Preheat oven to 325 degrees.
2. In a large bowl, add flour, no salt baking powder, and cinnamon. Whisk together until mixed.
3. Beat eggs, oil, vanilla, applesauce, and sugar together by hand in a large bowl or using a stand mixer until everything is well combined.
4. Add dry ingredients to the creamed mixture and beat well.
5. Fold in zucchini until well combined. Pour batter into prepared pans.

6. Bake for 40 to 60 minutes, or until a tester inserted in the center comes out clean.
7. Cool in pan on a wire rack for about 20 minutes. Remove loaf and let cool completely on the rack before attempting to cut.

27. Low Sodium Sloppy Joe
Prep Time: 00 Minutes

Cook Time: 23 Minutes

Servings: 4

Ingredients

- 2 teaspoons of dried minced onion
- 1/2 teaspoon of garlic powder
- 1/2 teaspoon of ground dried mustard
- 1/4 teaspoon of salt free chili powder
- 1/4 teaspoon of black pepper
- 1 pound of lean ground beef
- 1/2 cup of water
- 1 and 1/2 teaspoons of cider vinegar
- 1 cup no salt added ketchup

Instructions

1. In a large bowl add garlic powder, ground dried mustard, salt-free chili powder, black pepper, water, cider vinegar, and ketchup. Wisk together until combine and set aside.
2. Place ground beef and dried minced onion into a large nonstick skillet over medium heat until beef is brown. Be sure to break up the beef into small chunks.
3. Add your bowl of ingredients to the beef and onions. Bring to a gentle boil.
4. Once boiling, reduce heat to low and simmer for 10-15 minutes. Stir occasionally.

28. Low Sodium Pork Tenderloin with Apples
Prep Time: 15 Minutes

Cook Time: 25 Minutes

Servings: 4

Ingredients

- 1 pound of pork tenderloin, cut into pieces
- 1 1/2 tablespoons of curry powder
- 1 tablespoon of extra-virgin olive oil
- 2 cups of chopped yellow onions
- 2 cups of apple cider, divided
- 1 target apple, peeled, seeded, and cut into chunks
- 1 tablespoon of cornstarch

Instructions

1. Season the pork tenderloin with curry powder and let stand anywhere from15 minutes to overnight. (Refrigerate covered in saranwrap if letting stand overnight)
2. In a large, heavy skillet, heat the olive oil over medium-high heat. Add the tenderloin and cook, turning once, until browned on both sides, about 5 to 10 minutes. Remove the meat from the skillet and set it aside. Don't remove the juice from the pan!
3. Place the onions in the skillet and saute to tender. Add 1 and 1/2 cups of the apple cider, reduce heat and simmer until the liquid has reduced by half.

4. Add the chopped apple, cornstarch, and the remaining 1/2 cup cider. Stir and simmer while the sauce thickens, about 2 minutes.
5. Return the tenderloin to the skillet and simmer for the final 5 minutes.

29. Low Sodium Granola Muffins
Prep Time: 25 Minutes

Cook Time: 00 Minutes

Servings: 12

Ingredients

For The Muffins

- 1/2 cup of granulated sugar
- 2 large eggs, at room temperature
- 1/2 cup of canola or vegetable oil
- 2 teaspoons of vanilla extract
- 1 1/2 cups of bread flour
- 1 1/2 teaspoons of sodium-free baking powder
- 1 cup of unsalted granola
- 3/4 cup of buttermilk

For The Topping

- 1 cup of unsalted granola
- 2 tablespoons of brown sugar
- 1 tablespoon of all-purpose flour
- 2 tablespoons of unsalted butter, melted
- 1/4 teaspoon of cinnamon

Instructions

1. Preheat your oven to 350 degrees. Prepare your muffin tin by spray with a nonstick that contains flour or by lining them with paper liners.

2. In a bowl, whisk together the flour, granola, and sodium-free baking powder, set aside.
3. In a large bowl, whisk together the eggs and sugar until fluffy and pale. Next, add oil and vanilla, whisk to combine.
4. Add the dry ingredients along with the buttermilk to the egg/sugar/oil/vanilla mixture. Mix until just combined.
5. Fill prepared muffin tins evenly with batter. Set aside.
6. In a small bowl, stir together the ingredients for the topping. Sprinkle evenly on top of each individual muffin.
7. Bake at 350 degrees for about 20 minutes, or until a toothpick inserted into the middle of one of the center muffins comes out clean.
8. Allow muffins to cool in the pan, and after 5 minutes (or when they're cool enough to handle) transfer them to a wire rack to cool.

30. Low Sodium Thai Peanut Chicken

Prep Time: 00 Minutes

Cook Time: 30 Minutes

Servings: 4

Ingredients

- 1/2 cup of a low sodium peanut butter
- 3/4 cup of water
- 2 tablespoons of balsamic vinegar
- 1 tablespoon of minced garlic
- 1 tablespoon of fresh lemon juice
- 1.5 pounds of boneless, skinless chicken breast, cut into 1" pieces
- 1 red bell pepper, diced
- 1 medium onion, diced
- 1/2 cup of unsalted peanuts, rough chopped
- 1 1/2 cup of carrots, finely chopped
- 1/2 teaspoon of crushed red pepper flakes, optional
- 1 tablespoon of olive oil

Instructions

1. In a small mixing bowl, whisk together the peanut butter, balsamic vinegar, garlic, lemon juice, and water until fully blended to create your sauce. Set aside.
2. In a sauté pan, cook the vegetables in olive oil until translucent, and remove from the pan and set aside.
3. Using the same sauté pan, cook the chicken and peanuts in the oil until the chicken is cooked through.

Remember to flip your pieces of chicken so each side gets a nice brown sear.

4. While you are cooking your chicken, start preparing your side dish of choice by boiling your rice or pasta.
5. When the chicken has reached an internal temperature of 165 degrees, add your vegetables and peanut sauce to the pan. Let simmer over medium-low heat for 10-15 minutes, stirring occasionally.
6. Plate your Thai peanut chicken with your rice (or pasta) and dust the finished dish with red pepper flakes and chopped peanuts.